THE HEALTHY WOMAN: INSIDE AND OUT

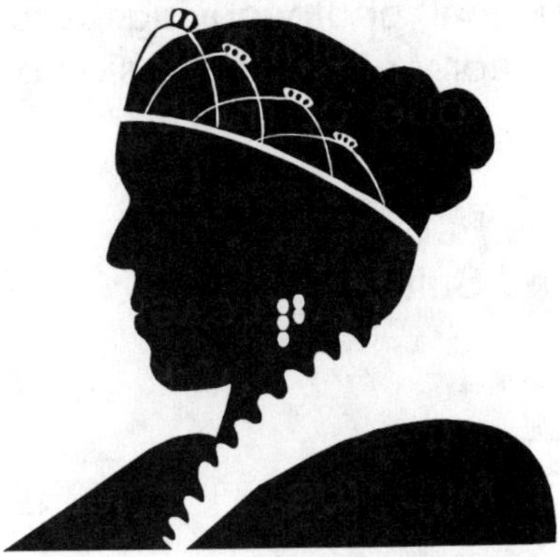

By
Adele J. Foster

Aquarius Creations Publishing
TEXAS

Published by
Aquarius Creations Publishing
2600 Preston Road Suite 1324
Plano, TX 75093

ISBN:1-928673-05-8

Printed in the United States of America

"For I am the Lord that health thee"

Exodus 15:26

ACKNOWLEDGEMENTS

I like to acknowledge the following individuals and organizations for their support and encouragement during this laboring process.

First and foremost, I like to thank God for discernment and vision. Without Him this book would still be in the laboring process waiting to be born.

Mark Muhammad of Powerhouse Speakers who booked a speaking engagement for me in Harrisburg, PA. Because of this engagement I became pregnant with *The Healthy Woman: Inside and Out.*

Bridgett Martin and her school district for having me as their Keynote Speaker in Harrisburg, PA on April 14, 2001. The Mother's, Daughter's and Sister-friend's Motivation and Empowerment Conference truly made this laboring process a pleasure.

Robert E. Criner, thank you for your encouraging words, post-cards, vision, support and most of all allowing Spirit to speak to you about The Healthy Woman: Inside and out.

Edwina T. Frazier, for recognizing that this book needed more than just a rah rah, but it also

needed action that could help the reader begin to become a healthy person.

Greeba D. Foster, my mother, for believing that I could do anything that I set my mind to and also for her contribution of "*Mighty Women of God*"

To my son, Al-Tariq Foster, who help me to understand what motherhood was all about.

To my loving and supportive husband, Tony D. Abel who made the final stages of this laboring worth while.

To Sanyu Barnicoat and Jean McDonald for agreeing to be my publicity in addition to being a true support system in my life.

To Delores Eleazer, a true sister who went for the ride and supported me throughout the process. Thank you!

And

To all the women, who I know and believe can become Healthy Women: Inside and Out because inside of you there is a positive spirit waiting to be born.

TABLE OF CONTENTS

Notes
At the end of this book are blank pages, please use them to journalize your thoughts, ideas, emotions, etc.

You will find it to be a healthy as well as a useful tool in releasing anything that is not good.

INTRODUCTION

In a conversation with my sister, she compliments me by saying I am a Mighty Woman of God. I like to pass that on today and tell you that you are mighty mothers, daughters, and sister-friends of God. Now say out loud, ***"I Am A Mighty Woman of God!"*** You see the word ***Mighty*** has power and as mighty mothers, daughters and sister-friends you have a toolbox of power. The power that you have can rule the world and make you **The Healthy Woman: Inside and Out.** This book is about becoming ***"The Healthy Woman: Inside and Out.***

In the beginning I mentioned a toolbox of power that you possess. Let us briefly explore what's inside that tool-box that will empower you to conquer your world. I will use the acronym **SLEEP** to help define the tools in your box. Sleep can cause peacefulness within your life. It can raise you above the drama and the nightmares and cause you to be calm and serene. **S-L-E-E-P**, **S** for Spirituality, **L** for Love and Family, **E** for Education, **E** for Emotions and **P** for Psychology. Each of us possess these tools but we may not know how to use them.

Let's start with the first letter, **S** for Spirituality. It is the foundation that keeps us grounded. It is having faith and knowing that whatever we chose to have is possible.

Inside each one of us lays a Spiritual foundation just waiting to be explored. Unfortunately, at an early age we are taught such words as don't, can't won't, no and have been conditioned to believe that little girls that soon grow-up and become adults are to respond accordingly.

I remember my grandmother saying, *"Now as a young lady you can not hop a fence or climb a tree. Young ladies are supposed to carry themselves in a certain way. You will be proper, prim and poise."* I never understood why because I enjoyed hopping fences and climbing trees, it was at those times I felt free, besides it didn't make me less of a woman.

My mother and father would tell us, *"What goes on in the household stays in the household."* Maybe your parents told you the same thing. So therefore, we grow up and become stingy. We don't want to share. We say things like, *"I don't want anyone to know my business."* What business? Your business is somebody business because somebody has gone through what you have been through. I recall having a conversation with a friend who said, *"Women should never go buy a car or furniture without a man."* That is some illogical thinking. With those beliefs and others we begin to lose sight of what is inside speaking to us and we learn to listen to those individuals who believe they know what's right for us. Let's put them away forever and begin to listen to that inner spirit that says, "*Whatever we want, need, or desire can be obtained.*

The Bible talks about having FAITH as small as a mustard seed and being able to say to a mountain move and it shall be moved. (Mat. 17:20) That's some strong Faith. Well, I am here to tell you, mothers, daughters, and sister-friends, inside of you live that same kind of Faith. The minute you bring it to the surface, change will take place.

Change takes place when you get sick and tried of being sick and tried. It takes place when you get tired of doing the same thing day in and day out. It takes place when you get tired of those temporary fixes. It takes place when your emotional bank balance becomes overdrawn. It takes place when you have grounded yourself spiritually and began having the FAITH knowing that whatever you ask for it shall be given to you. That's what happens to the Healthy Woman: Inside and Out.

Now let's take a look at the **L** for love and family. If you could fall in love with the most wonderful person in the world, what are some of the things you would do with that person? As I ponder over that question, I realized that we as mothers, daughters, and sisterfriends are always in search of the one thing that makes us happy, contented and satisfied. Not realizing that we have been looking for love in all the wrong places. The search or the journey that we take ourselves through is within us. We don't need to go looking on the outside for what exist on the inside. We are equipped with some powerful tools.

Sue Patton Theole states in her book, *The Courage To Be Yourself* that, *"Without an awareness of ourself, the courage to express who we are, and the willingness to experience the discomfort and exhilaration that follows, we are not truly living. We are existing merely as mirrors, reflecting other people's lives. Until we are able to become our unique and beautiful (and, sometimes, ugly and mundane) selves, we cannot truly love either ourselves or others and love is what life is all about."*

Hmm...If you could fall in love with the most wonderful person in the world.... let me tell you the most wonderful person in the world is **YOU!**

When was the last time you looked in the mirror and said, I love you? Have you loved you lately? Today, right now I give you permission to give yourself a great big hug. Come on, put this book down and hug yourself. Now, didn't that feel good? Have you kissed you lately? Again, I give you permission to kiss yourself. Come on take your hand and give yourself a kiss.

Remember the song by Chaka Kahn which was later sung by Whitney Houston, *"I'm Every Woman?"* Well you are, you're the mother, the daughter, the sister, the girlfriend, the wife, the career woman and this list goes on. That's why it is so important to love yourself from the inside so that you can have an abundance of love to come flowing to the outside. The love that will come pouring out will be an overflow to the family and it is what helps to keep the family together.

As the mother you are the matriarch, you are the head and not the tail. As the daughter you are the helper and as the sisterfriend, you are the support system. With all three systems in place you help keep the family as a unit. Therefore, it is important to understand that it takes a village to raise a family and in case no one ever told you, the backbone in the village are the women.

So how do we continue to keep ourselves spiritually grounded and keep loving ourselves from the inside out so that it can cause an overflow in the family? Well that leads us right into the next letter of the acronym, **E** for Education. It is so important that we keep feeding our spiritual souls with the right information. It is studying the giants who paved the path: like Rosa Parks who refused to move and knowing that the first black millionaire was a woman by the name of Madam C.J. Walker and reading and studying the life and times of Mary McCloud Bethune just to name a few. They paved the path so we no longer have to be Pathfinders but Trailblazers.

Mothers follow the path that has been opened for you. Daughters open yourself up to receive the wisdom of this earth and sisterfriends continue to be the support system that is very much needed and for all of you, do not allow yourself to be taken into the next letter E called ***E***motions.

You see as women, we tend to walk around with PMS (Poor Me Syndrome.) Sue Patton Theole writes in her book, _The Courage To Be Yourself_, *"women have a deep need for emotional connectedness and intimacy. That is not all bad. In fact this desire is what makes us such wonderful lovers, friends and mothers. But when that need is not balanced with the need to be our own person, we can become emotionally dependent, losing sight of ourselves and all our capabilities."*

I don't know about you but for me whenever I felt disconnected I would tell myself I was fine. I recall a time that I had to do a speech and a week before I had to deliver that speech I became depressed. I would tell people who were close to me how depressed I was feeling. When people would ask me how I was doing? I would say fine and I was fine; I was **F**RUSTRATED, **I**NSECURE, **N**EROTIC and **E**MOTIONAL. I was real fine. I began to psychologically realize what I was doing. I was allowing my thoughts to control my emotions. And if I could tell myself I was depressed, I could also write another script that says, I am blessed. What script are you writing today? A sure tool that worked for me was to take every negative and turn it into a positive. That meant I had to pay close attention to what I was speaking and thinking. By doing this I created an environment to empower myself. Therefore, I did not have to be emotionally dependent on negativity. Instead, I became really **FINE**; (after self-empowerment), I was **F**aithful, **I**ndependent, **N**ourished (by God's blessings) and **E**ducated (full of knowledge).

Proverbs tell us that, *"As a man thinketh, so is he..." (Proverbs 23:7)* If we begin to think positive thoughts we will not have room for those negative emotions. Proverbs also tells us that *"death and life are in the power of the tongue."* (Proverbs 18:21) So what are you speaking today? Try applying some psychological techniques in your life by using affirmations, such as:

- I deserve to be love;
- I am in control of myself;
- I have the right to be happy;
- I deserve to have all that I desire.

Begin to write your own affirmations. Read them daily, say them daily. Study them until you transform into the Healthy Woman: Inside and Out.

SPIRITUALITY

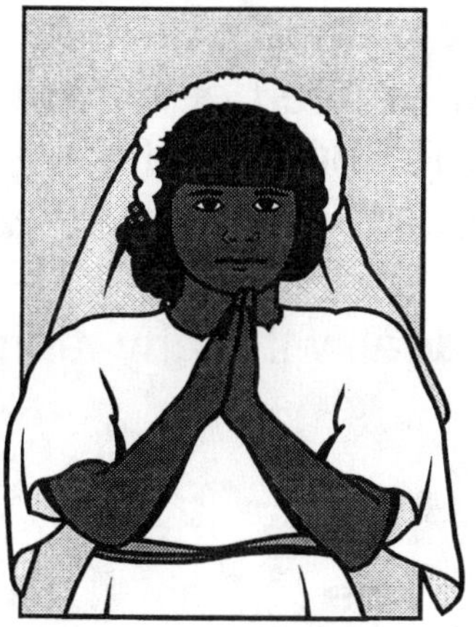

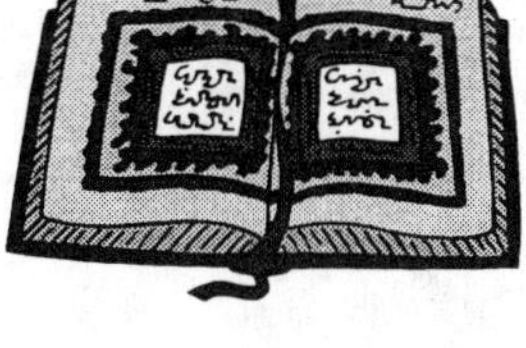

SPIRITUALITY

"I can do all things through Christ which strengthen me."
Phil 4:13

Becoming the healthy woman inside and out is a process. So where do you start? I believe that as women we should ground ourselves spiritually. When I think about the trials and tribulations that I have been through, I know that the one thing that kept me going was the Word. So right now, I want to tell you to *"WORD UP!"* The word will help you deal with any and all situations.

"I can do all things through Christ who strengthens me." (Phil. 4:13) Yes, you can. Believing and trusting that Christ is your energy source can cause a wonderful transformation in your life. Fear will be eliminated, doubt will disappear, discouragement will no longer exist and loneliness will not be a state of mind.

Spirituality will help you in conquering any storms. It will truly keep you with peace of mind and will put you on the path of wholeness. There is no storm you can not weather when you allow spirituality into your life. Developing a relationship with the Creator will allow you to become whole and complete.

In my life I have been faced with many challenges but I discovered throughout the Bible there was a scripture for every challenge I was facing. So for every stronghold that tries to invade my world, I know that God has a word to turn it around.

Proverbs teaches us to:

> *Trust in the Lord with all thine heart; and lean not unto thine own understanding. In all thy*

ways acknowledge Him, and
He shall direct thy path.
Proverbs 3:5-6

"Trust in the Lord with all thine heart." Trusting God is really a very simple process but most of the time we complicate it by allowing the flesh to take control and then we question why?

"Lean not unto thine own understanding." Some of us as women are always trying figure things out, so we can fix it. If we practice giving God the control we would find life much easier and learn that there is nothing too great or too small that God can't fix.

"In all thy ways acknowledge Him." Acknowledge Him in prayer, in good times, and in bad times. Give Him the Honor, the Glory, and the Praise.

"He shall direct thy path." Life will be a bright ball of sunshine, there will be

some rain but with God directing our paths we can't go wrong.

<u>Try this on:</u>
Perhaps you are at a time in your life where there seems to be trouble all around you. You keep searching for a way out but there seems to be no where to go. Begin to start praying and asking God for the answer to your problem.

After you have lift your problems up in pray, perhaps you might want to write a letter to God defining all the good things that you would like to have happen for you in your life.

The answer may come to you in a dream, or in the next day or two.

The one thing that I can promise you is God does answer prayers. Just ask

Him for discernment to be able to hear, see, and act on the answer.

Often our problem is not that we don't hear God but we fail to respond in obedience. The bible says *it's not hearers only of the word who will be blessed but the doers.* Romans 2:13

LOVE AND FAMILY

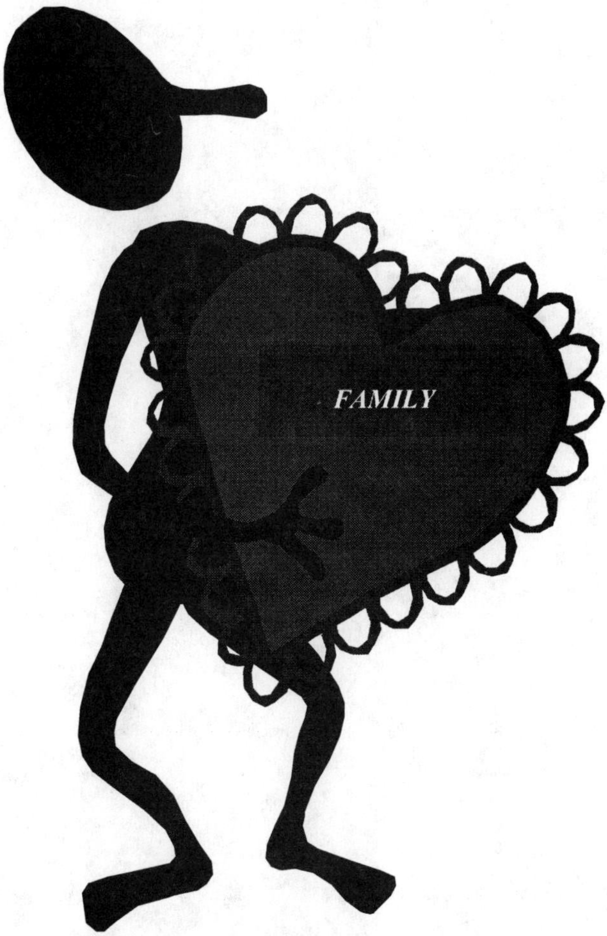

LOVE AND FAMILY

"All things work together for good to them that love God…."
Romans 8:28

Love

As women we tend to give our love away. We give it to our children, our husband/significant other, our family, and friends and we don't have enough left over to give to ourselves.

Love is a very vital source of our life. But as women, we are nurturers. We take care of everyone but ourselves. Those few times we dare to do something for ourselves; guilt sets in. We think we're being selfish. We even give ourselves excuses, as though we don't deserve to be pampered and cared for. Not all of us fit into this category some of us have learned the value of looking out for number one first. If you consistently take time for yourself…..you go girl! But if you don't read on.

If I were to tell you to sit in silence for five minutes, could you? That five minutes might feel like five hours, that's because we believe we must be busy at all times. Busy cleaning the house, taking care of the family, friends, cooking, working the job, busy, busy, busy**...** **STOP!** Take time for youself.

In the book *Sacred Pampering Principles*, Debrena Jackson Gandy states the question, *"What kind of things would you do if you were in love with the most wonderful person in the world?"*

Take a moment and concentrate on that question. Now write all the wonderful things that you would do with that person.

1. ______________________________

2. ______________________________

3. ______________________________

4. ______________________________

5. ______________________________

6. ______________________________

7. _______________________________

8. _______________________________

Did you get a warm fuzzy feeling just thinking and writing all the wonderful things that you would do with that person? You probably even visualize the person to whom you would be sharing those moments with. The good feeling that you were experiencing can be transferred to yourself, all those wonderful things that you would do with someone else can be can be done for yourself.

That's the point that Debrena was making. The most wonderful person in the world is you! And if you could do those things with someone else then why can't you begin doing them for yourself.

I have discovered that the inner love that I have for myself created an abundance of love that I could give to everyone else and still have enough room to love myself.

Society has truly conditioned us as little girls not to think too highly of ourselves. An example of this is:

Ever remember as a little girl if you should act or think that you were cute, you would be labeled as being conceited? In my day, mothers cautioned us not to show off. Children were supposed to be seen but not heard. So we suppress our thoughts of being cute or became conscious of whether we were demonstrating anything that would make others think that we were acting in such a way. It doesn't surprise me that many of us grew up with self-esteem issues.

Can you recall a time when you really felt good about yourself? You felt so good about yourself that you could feel it deep within. The experience that was taking place on the inside caused an outwardly glow and everyone you met could feel and see the effect of your beauty within. That feeling can be captured over and over again, if we learn how to apply those feelings without bringing along the baggage. The baggage is what intoxicates our mind, our soul, our body and our spirit. The sad part about it is that we allow it to take up space and we don't ask it to pay rent. There is a price that we pay when we allow negativity to invade our space. It costs us love, health, vitality, peace, understanding, wisdom and knowledge. It stunts our growth and robs us of the opportunity to truly experience the fullness of life.

As women loving ourselves first is so important in our lives that we can't afford to be without it. Once we arrive at the level of loving ourselves there is an abundance of overflowing love we can pass on to the family.

Family

As women, family is so important to us; whether it is our immediate family or the family we adopted. We want them to constantly know that our love is everlasting and we show it by what we say and what we do, and how we care for them. The beauty about this is receiving it back and the acceptance is so gratifying, that we do not want to lose those feelings. We are instructed by God to keep the family together and therefore the village is formed. Keeping all things in place, children, husband and others that we have included in the family. Therefore in the mist of doing all of that and more for the family we must be careful not to lose sight of who we are.

As women we believe in taking care of the family without letting anyone know how we really feel inside. Our inside suffers for the satisfaction of healing the family and no one seems to recognize that we need that same healing too. That rest would do us good but because of the need to please others we keep going like an Eveready battery. Somehow we fail to recognize that the energy is low and we have to replenish that which was taken away or else an imbalance of the mind, body, soul and spirit occurs. Our level of love for the family becomes an irritant emotion that no one understands. We began to project our inward emotions to the family. This may be done through criticism believing that no can do things or know things the way we do. This is when the love for the family becomes stagnant. Ever notice that other family members take your lead? If you criticize, they are critical; if you withhold your love and not give, they are selfish. Let's stop and think about what is happening, they are only giving to you what you are reflecting about yourself.

Before I began to educate myself on those emotional turmoils in my life, I thought it was just a passing phase, it will eventually go away. Nothing goes away by itself and if something is not done you can lose sight of the family and yourself. So you see it is so vital that love begin inwardly, because we have a whole family as well as a village that respects and depend on our strength. They see us as the matriarch. Look at life today, if daddy leaves, things are semi-okay, (not saying that it is okay for daddy to leave); but if mama leaves there is destruction. What can we do? How do we survive? You see the role of the mother, who is also the daughter, as well as the sister girlfriend is so important. We can not afford to be weakened or be encamped by anything that is not positive.

Try this on:

In the morning when you wake-up, go straight to a mirror and say, *"I LOVE YOU"* ten times. Then give yourself a hug to embrace what God has in store for you today.

Or try this:

Write or say:

I love you because _____________.

Then look in the mirror and think of all the things you love/like about yourself. Turn them into verbal affirmations and say them to yourself.

Example:
I love you because you're funny. I am a humors person. I feel good when I make myself and others laugh.

I love you because you're quiet. I am a quiet person. I often see what others do not because I take the time to observe my surroundings.

EDUCATION

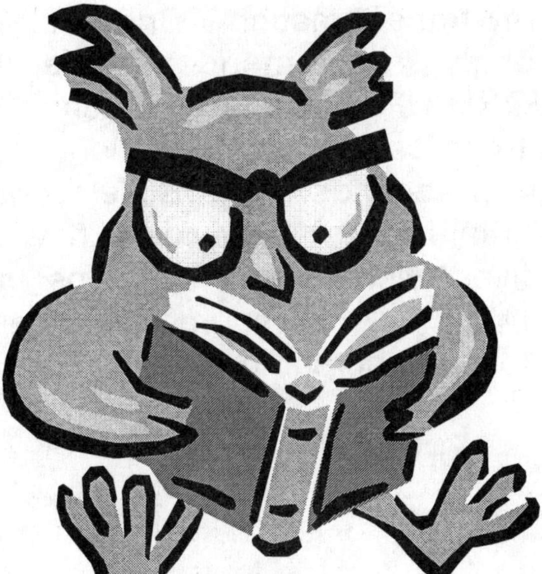

EDUCATION

"My people will perish for the lack of knowledge...
Proverbs 29:18

I am an avid reader and I truly believe reading can be **fun**damental. I remember when I was going through my transformation stages of becoming a healthy woman there were certain books I had to read and own. I did not just read those books but I pulled out of those books certain principles that I could apply to my daily life that would help me in my transformation. One book that I strongly recommend is the Bible (WORD UP) there is so much in there that can cause transformation to happen in seconds. The Bible feeds our spiritual beings, it provides knowledge; it gives wisdom and develops understanding. It's the source that connects us to God and our inner self.

Another form of educating ourselves is finding mentors who can guide you in the process of transforming into the healthy woman inside and out. Studying the giants such as Mary Kay Ashly, Oprah Winfrey, Hillary Clinton, Iyanla Vanzant, Louise Hay, Terri Williams, Susan Taylor and Dottie Walters, these are just a few women who paved a path for me. I am sure that if you dig deeply you can come up with some individuals who had a great impact on your life. Individuals you have studied or would like to study because they have done something that you would like to do. Think for a second who are they? What is it that they did and how did they do it? Once you have the answer all you have to do is trail the blaze because they have already paved the path. We have the most powerful tool in the world. It is our mind and if we feed it properly we can achieve far beyond our means. One thing about our mind is it does not know the difference between the real and the imagined. So therefore, we can create whatever we choose and make it a possibility. I say create positive and exciting things. Life is fun, treat it that way. All the drama, issues, and baggage that we carry around is only a script that we have written in our head. Believe it or not we can rewrite the script, because we are in control. Educating ourselves to do this is a process that can be done.

Remember the commercial that stated:

> *"A Mind is a Terrible Thing to Waste?"*

So why are you wasting what God has given you? *God has not given you a spirit of fear* (2Tim. 1:7), so release any fear and use the power that God has given to create a sound mind. With a sound mind you can pour so much inside of you, that makes you positive, strong, and healthy.

RENEW YOUR MIND

> *"Be not conformed to this*
> *world; but be ye transformed*
> *by the renewing of your mind."*
> (Romans 12:2)

Education is such an important factor in becoming a Healthy Woman. The better educated we are the least likely we will fall into pitfalls and valleys.

Even though education is number three in the process, it is a vital tool to have.

It is what makes us soar like giants or crawl like ants. Through education we can become fully aware of who we are, and where we are and where we can go.

Try this on:

Get a highlighter and a Bible.

Read your Bible first thing in the morning and just before you go to bed at night. As you are reading, highlight anything that you can apply in your new journey to becoming a Healthy Woman.

Example:

In my Bible, I have highlighted:

"For I am the Lord that healeth thee..." Ex. 15:26

How do I apply it?

When adversity comes up against my mind, my body, my soul, or my spirit, I can react by reminding myself that I serve a God who heals. So I speak it out loud:

"I SERVE A GOD THAT HEALS MY MIND, MY BODY, MY SOUL AND MY SPIRIT."

EMOTIONS

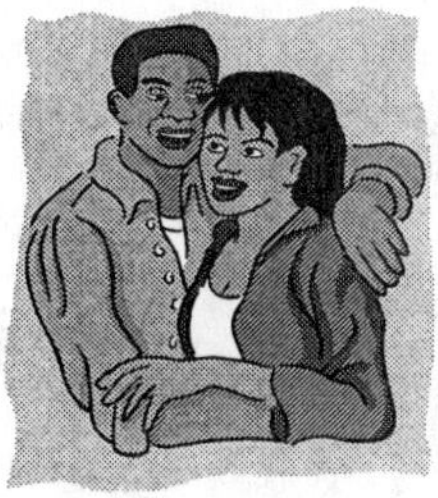

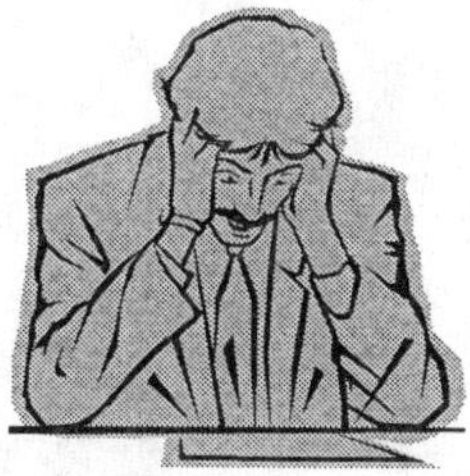

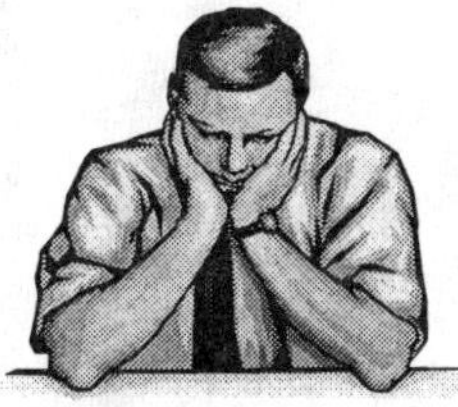

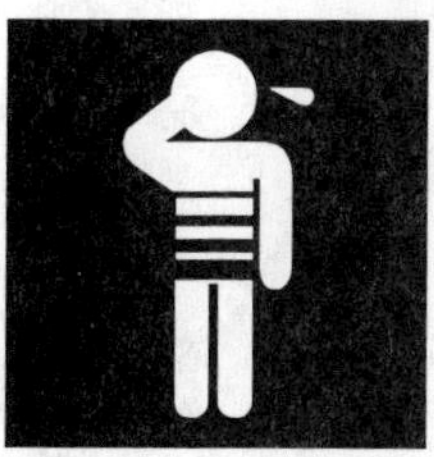

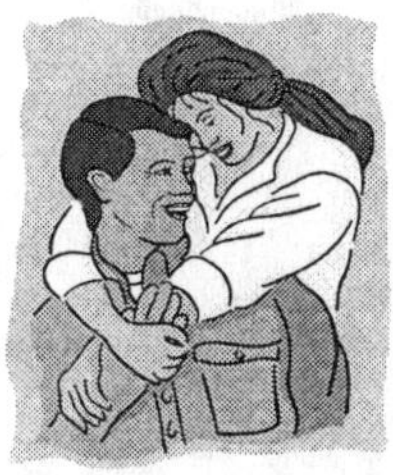

EMOTIONS

"For God hath not given us the spirit of fear: but of power, and of love, and of a sound mind."
2Tim. 1:7

Emotions, they make us happy, they create joy, they make us cry, they make us sad, they make us confused, they cause disappointment as well as frustration. Emotions, where do they come from? How can we control them?

As women we go through so many emotional changes that we sometimes do not understand ourselves nor what we are going through. We even give our emotional changes names—how interesting. But the fact is if we could educate ourselves to the imbalances that our insides are experiencing, then we will become equipped to deal with those emotions that we are feeling from time to time.

I remember the first time I experienced pre-menstrual syndrome (I was in my late 20's) I felt as though my nerves were under attack. The least little thing that someone said to me would strike a nerve, but it did not just strike one nerve, it struck many nerves and I was out of control. Remember in the last chapter, I talked about education? I educated myself to the chemical imbalances in my life; I began to understand and even recognize when pre-menstrual syndrome wanted to invade my body. Therefore I was able to take back my control and not give it away.

Another form of an emotional state is dishonesty. Part of becoming the healthy woman: inside and out requires that you are honest with yourself.

When you are honest with yourself than you can be honest with others.

The most volatile of emotions is fear. Fear will keep us from moving and saying exactly how we feel. We harbor such fears of hurting someone else, fear of stepping out on FAITH. While inside we are suffering because we refuse to express how we feel, what we feel and what we are going through. We, as women, sometime tend to be people pleasers, and the drama queen in us comes to life when we are not certain of how to express what we are feeling. But what we fail to realize is that others are not mind readers, and the only person we are in control of, is ourselves. We can not control others thoughts, actions or behaviors. Even though we would like to, we must realize that if we let it go, there could be less baggage to carry. The baggage we chose to carry causes a lot of our emotional states. You see, we not only carry our own baggage, but we carry our friends' as well as strangers' issues. You got to release it, let it go, don't own it, it's not yours.

When I was a teenager, strangers would come up to me and tell me their problems. I never said anything back to them I would just listen. My sister would ask me did I know these strangers and secondly, why were they telling me their business? At the time, I just answered her by saying, "I don't know." As I became older, I realized that they no longer wanted to bear their pain, anxiety, and anguish; therefore, telling it to someone they didn't know meant they would not have to hear it again. It's like seeking God in a quiet place and He lifts those burdens off your shoulders and you walk away with peace of mind. *(Let go, let God!)*

Try this on:

Say exactly how you feel.
Talk to a tape recorder and record everything that you are feeling inside.

OR……

Write a letter to yourself expressing those inner emotions.

Put them aside for a day or two and then re-listen or re-read what you said or wrote, then discard it. This process will help you to cleanse your inner spirit as well as create a new beginning.

PSYCHOLOGY

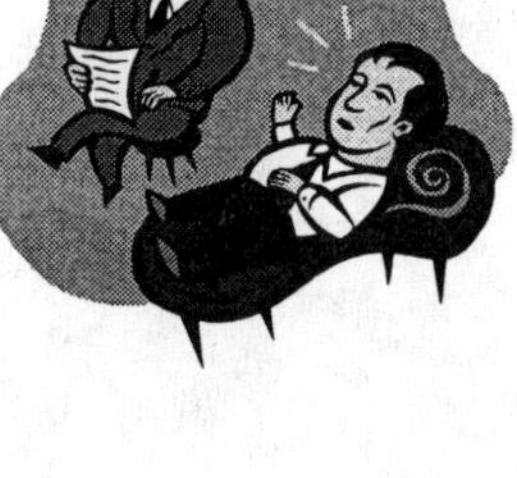

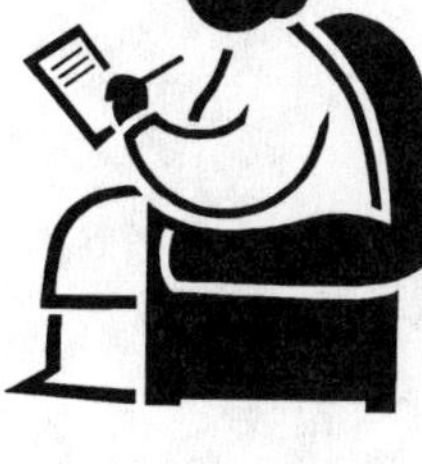

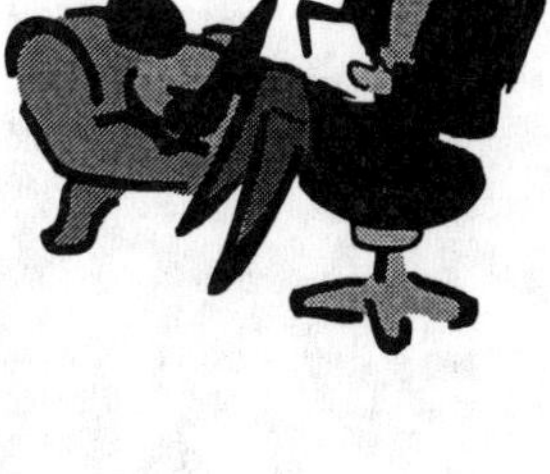

PSYCHOLOGY

"Death and life is in the power of the tongue…"
Proverbs 18:21

Psychologically speaking we as women write so many stories. We write a story about ourselves, we write a story about our parents, we write a story about our mates, our children, jobs, household and this list can continue. The stories we write, we believe. It has become a part of our **DNA**. Therefore no one can tell us anything different about the story (ies) we have written. The truth of the matter is we walk around with these stories and they become our possessions. That's right we own those stories, they belong to us, and we don't want anyone to take them.

HER STORY

An old acquaintance of mine has psychologically put herself in bondage .

She writes a story that goes like this:

> *"If my mother had not died and left me when I was a little girl; If my father had not taken up with another family and left my aunt to raise me; perhaps my life would be different. And now that I am 42 years old; I know people who can help me but they won't, even though I would do the same for them. My life will never get any better because of what I have experience."*

The story that she has written, she is living, believing and speaking. It has become part of her database. It is what I call **GIGO.** Garbage In; Garbage Out. Until she rewrites her story that bondage will remain a part of her database.

In order to create a healthy environment we have to learn to stop writing those never ending stories. Liz Lisker, a trainer and consultant says it well. She states:

"Our brains are like computers— programmed by our culture, family, peers, and our own inborn talents and temperament. Some of that programming may not be "user friendly". *In fact, many of us are likely to have picked up viruses along the way. Our programming affects our health, relationships, creativity, happiness, and our professional and personal success. Most of our programming, however is out of our awareness, installed in us as children, by parents, teachers, social upbringing, and the media long before we could be aware of how it would impact our lives or realized we had choices. We*

were imprinted to be believers – not thinkers. Just as you can re-program your computer, you can re-program your brain so it totally supports you."

MY STORY

I enjoy psychology and am always curious about "what makes people tick?". I began to study and observe us as women. Starting with myself as the first subject. I found many things about me that I was not pleased about. Were they right or wrong? I will say that they were only learning processes, self-discoveries and tools that can be used to create change. As you go through your process of self-discovery you may say the same thing.

The things that I discovered that I did not like about myself were the stories that I had written and believed.

Some of my stories started as early as childhood and I carried them with me. Other stories began when I became an adult and thought that something must be wrong with me if things did not go a certain way.

A couple of insights about myself; I was shy (possibly caused by low self-esteem). I was not smart (this stem from early childhood). Nobody loves me; I'm too skinny. There's a pattern forming, sounds familiar? I am sure you can add to the above because most of the time as we grow into womanhood we tend to look for flaws and allow it to create our world.

> *"As a man thinketh in his heart, so is he."*
> (Proverbs 23:7)

You see those things that we think about ourselves we believe, not only do we believe it, we become it.

Our thoughts are so powerful that it creates a world of whatever we chose to live. Ever notice how easy it is to believe that which is negative about ourselves, about the people we surround ourselves with, about the world? What would happen if we replace each negative thought with a positive one? Begin to imagine the possibilities of joy, happiness, peace of mind, relaxation. This does exist if you allow it.

"*Death and life is in the power of the tongue*" Proverbs 18:21

I am firm believer that we create our lives by what we speak. If we take some time and listen to those words that are form out of our mouths, we might be surprised how we are channeling it into our world. Whatever happens in life has already taken place before. Why? Because we spoke it which allowed us to believe it. Therefore it should not be a surprise when it shows up. But often it is a surprise because we do not hear those things in which we speak into existence. We just say them for the moment , not realizing that it is creating our world.

Try this on:

As you go through your day use affirmations that will empower you. Such as:

I am a Mighty Woman of God.

I can do all things through Christ who strengthens me.

I am whole, healthy and complete.

Write some positive affirmations of your own.

My own affirmations:

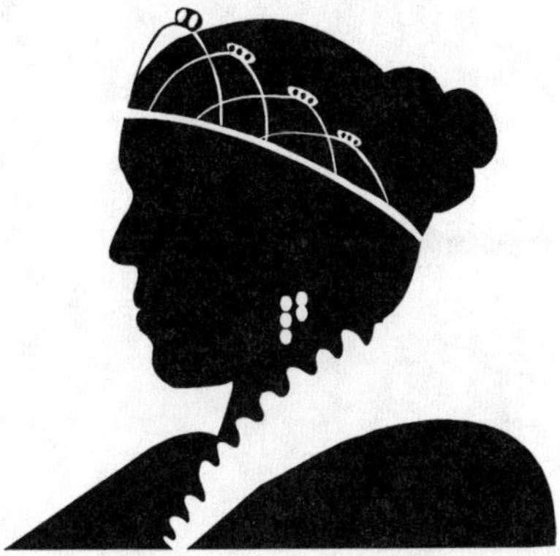

TOOLS FOR BECOMING THE HEALTHY WOMAN: INSIDE AND OUT

Daily
Mediation and Affirmations
A Healing Process for
The Mind, Body, Soul and Spirit

TOOLS FOR BECOMING THE HEALTHY WOMAN: INSIDE AND OUT

Becoming a healthy woman is a process. It requires daily communication with your spiritual self. That means taking time for mediation and silence.

It requires a time to love yourself and replenish what you have given away.

It requires gaining a sense of knowledge to help you in your struggles.

It requires absolute control over your emotions even when hormonal nature wants to get in the way.

It requires utilization of our psychological intuition. So that we can battle any journey that is before us. It's remembering that:

"No weapons formed against thee shall propser..."

Isaiah 54:17

In this section are tools to help you become the healthy woman inside and out. Use them to create change, to feel good, to create a **New World** that you thought never exist. Because you are a Mighty Woman of God and God does not fail us. He lifts us up and causes good things to happen.

TOOLS

The following are daily prayers, affirmations and mediation words to assist you in the journey of becoming a *Healthy Woman: Inside and Out.* Use them as you see fit in your journey, create some of your own. The idea to becoming healthy is grounding yourself spiritually, lovingly, emotionally, educationally, and psychologically. I believe these are some vital components to creating a healthy life.

TOOL # 1

This morning as you wake up start your day with a prayer.....

"Today, I will accomplish all that my Creator has in stored for me to accomplish. I thank the Creator for keeping me safely through out the night and awakening me with a sound mind. I am capable of achieving all that I set out to do today.

I AM A MIGHTY WOMAN OF GOD!

TOOL # 2

Sit for thirty minutes in silence. It is best to do this in the morning. I find mornings to be the most peaceful. The earth is awakening and you can hear God so clearly. Ask of God any question that you want an answer to, then sit in silence. The answer will come.

TOOL # 3

MIRROR IMAGE. I love the mirror because it never lies. Remember:

"Mirror, mirror on the wall…"

Go to your mirror and affirm out loud how much you love you. That's right, look straight into that mirror, hug you and say,

"I LOVE YOU!"

Say I Love You at least ten times. I promise you it will ingrain in your brain and you will never forget how much you love yourself. Nor will you accept anything less than the best because you are a precious gem.

ACTIVATE YOUR TOOLS

Tools 4-10 can be used as prayers, affirmations or can be written on pieces of paper and taped up where you can see and read them several times a day.

TOOL #4

Dear God,

Today, I will not place limitation on what it is that you will have me to accomplish. I will use all of the gifts and talents that you have given me along with sound wisdom that I receive directly from you. I know that I can do all things through you for you are my strength, my life and my salvation.

TOOL # 5

If at anytime you find yourself judging yourself or others, this prayer maybe a helpful reminder that judgment is just another form of negativity and it has no place in our lives.

Dear God,

Today, I will not judge for I know that when I judge others, I am only reflecting that of myself. I am wonderfully made because I am a product of you and therefore I am loved, I am healthy, I whole, I am complete, I am strong all because You have made me to be that way..

Thank you God, thank you.

TOOL # 6

"As a man thinketh in his heart; so is he...
Proverbs 23:

You are in control of your thoughts

Your thoughts create your environment

Your thoughts shape your world

What do you chose today?

I chose to think positive
I chose to have a healthy life
I chose to be happy

TOOL # 7

I am

All that I say,

All that I think,

And

All that I do

Therefore,

I will say positive words

I will think positive thoughts

I will do positive things.

TOOL # 8

NOW IS THE TIME

TO CHANGE

I

CHOSE TO CHANGE

FOR

THE BETTER

TOOL # 9

God

has given me the keys

to unlock many doors

I will go to the locks

and

use my keys wisely….

TOOL # 10

ME TIME

As I start my day, I know that

there is so much I want to accomplish

but I will first take time for me.

I will take 30-minutes to be in silence.

I will reverence my God for

assistance throughout this day.

I will constantly love myself.

I am full, whole and complete.

OH MIGHTY WOMEN OF GOD
By Greeba D. Foster

Oh Mighty Women of God. Speak out,
let your voices be heard.

Praise the Lord to all the world and
speak of His glorious word.

Oh Mighty Women of God, there's
much work to done. The world has
need of your knowledge about the Holy
One!

He came to this earth to save us from
our worldly sins. Open your ears with
honor and let the Savor in.

Oh Mighty Women of God, do you
know who you are?
Seek the Lord with all your heart. He's
not very far!

He always walking beside you; where ever you may go.

Tell Him about your trouble, tell Him about your woe.

God is a mighty spirit if you just let him in. He'll relieve you of your troubles, He'll free you from your sins.

God is a mighty healer, if you will just believe. Ask the Lord in earnest and blessings you will receive!

Oh Mighty Women of God, you were born for a reason

God blessed you with His love to be, a woman of all seasons.

Oh Mighty Women of God, Praise Him for all your worth.

Because of His plan for you; you were born upon this earth.

Speak out Oh Mighty Women of God.
Let your voices be heard. Praise the Lord
with all your heart and on earth you must
spread His Word!

Oh Mighty Women of God,
The world reaches out to you.

You are the mothers of life-long dreams.
Your hearts are filled to the utmost ex-
tremes.

The love of God surrounds you. The
beauty of earth is yours.

You're nature's bounty and wonder, as big
as all outdoors.

The outdoor world has serenity in trees of
green and gold. The majesty of tall moun-
tain peaks is a glory to behold!

Oh Mighty Women of God from you these
wonders unfold,
As you proclaim to all the world, the joy of
miracles untold.

Lift up your voices Oh Mighty Women of God, I give you peace from the Lord on High; from a place far beyond the magnificent sky. Thank Him for today, yesterday and tomorrow, for relief from pain, suffering and sorrow.

Oh Mighty Women of God, I lift you up to His Presence above. He bestows on you many blessings of abundant love.

Pray always for any reason. His grace and mercy are ever pleasing. Oh Mighty Women of God, man bows down to you, for you light up with spiritual bliss, the dark clouds in this world when things are amiss.

God has given you this wonderful gift, to represent Him and give the world a lift. Bow down Oh Mighty Women of God, humble yourselves before the Lord; for He will always bless you in wondrous great accord.

Speak out Oh Mighty Women of God, give the world God's word. In the light of His life, let His prophecies be heard.

THE JOURNEY CONTINUES....

Perhaps while we are taking our walk through life we will discover the peace and calmness of spirit. As spirit walks us to the next phase we learn the joys of what inner love can bring. Because of the inner love that we have found for ourselves we are able to spread an unconditional love that reaches and touches every family member. The essence of this flow does not stop because we continue to embrace education that allows our mind to absorb all the knowledge that will give us wisdom and understanding especially when those emotional attacks flair up and the stories start singing their songs. Psychologically we can become strong because we have learned to write a new song that will allow us to be…..

"THE HEALTHY WOMAN:
INSIDE AND OUT"

Suggested Readings

The Way I Am Now… Is Not The Way I'm Going To End Up!
By Edwina Frazier

Sacred Pampering Principles
By Debrena Jackson Gandy

All The Joy You Can Stand!
By Debrena Jackson Gandy

You Can Heal Your Life
By Louise Hay

The Courage To Be Yourself
(A Woman's Guide to Growing Beyond Emotional Dependence)
By Sue Patton

The Magic of Thinking Big
By David H. Schwartz, Ph.D

One Day My Soul Just Open Up
By Iyanla Vanzant

About The Author

ADELE J. FOSTER is an author, empowerment speaker, trainer, coach and a successful entrepreneur. Her extensive studies in business and marketing combined with her skills in communication have enabled her to educate, motivate and empower Fortune 500 companies, state agencies, entrepreneurs, work first recipients, housing residents, and head start parent groups causing them to break through self-impose barriers and operate at pcak performance. Adele specializes in training that emphasizes on creative approaches that causes transformation and realization of inner strength.

Over the last 10 years, Adele has been a consultant for the New Jersey Small Business Development Center, an entrepreneur trainer for the New Jersey Association of Women Business Owners, Essex County Wise Women Center, Adjunct Professor for Computer Information Systems for various colleges throughout New Jersey and at the same time she has been able to manage her own successful business. She has also been instrumental in empowering work first participants as well as homeless individuals and creating a difference in their lives.

With all the energy that Adele exemplifies it is no wonder why groups, companies and organizations that encounter Adele's overall aura can't wait to take the energy that she leaves them with and pass it on to others.

For more information on booksignings, lectures, and workshops,
Adele can be reached at
1-800-245-5880
or
E-mail: aquariuscreations@hotmail.com

SOON TO BE RELEASED
IN 2002

WOMEN OF GOD

THE HARVEST IS PLENTIFUL BUT THE LA-BORS ARE FEW

LOVE AT FIRST BYTE

STILL MORE ABOUT THE AUTHOR

She loves people. It makes her feel good when she has made a difference in someone's life.

She believes a positive attitude is the key to success in life.

She encourages everyone to THINK BIG because she knows that is what God wants for you.

She likes the butterfly because it is a symbol to be free.

She welcomes thoughts, ideas, comments, stories, and inspirational tidbits.

Send them to:

A.J. FOSTER & ASSOCIATES
2600 Preston Road, Ste. 1324
Plano, TX 75093
e-mail: aquariuscreations@hotmail.com

TOOLS FOR BECOMING A HEALTHY WOMAN

The Healthy Woman: Inside and Out Book
$14.95

The Healthy Woman: Inside and Out T-shirts
$15.00

Daily Affirmation and Meditation Cards
$7.50

The Healthy Woman: Inside and Out Key ring
$2.00

The Healthy Woman: Inside and Out Stone
$2.00

I Am A Mighty Woman of God Stone
$2.00

==============================

NAME________________________________

ADDRESS:____________________________
____

PHONE # ____________________________

E-MAIL ADDRESS: ____________________

_cash __check __money order _credit card
Credit card #__________________ exp. _____

Send to: 2600 Preston Road, Suite 1324,

NOTING MY WAY TO BECOMING A HEALTHY WOMAN

NOTES

NOTES

NOTES

NOTES

NOTES

NOTES

NOTES

NOTES